Low Carb

50 Top Low Carb Recipes for Weight Loss Secrets to Effortlessly Lose Your Weight Fast

By

Jamie Watson

ISBN-13: 978-1514801000
ISBN-10: 1514801000

Table of Contents

LOW CARB

INTRODUCTION

Welcome to this training for the Kindle! So you have decided to start a low carb diet and change your lifestyle. People, like you, opt this change for a number of reasons. Some do it for health reasons, some due to medical/dietary prescription, and some just want to lose weight and have better confidence in their bodies.

Yes – there are various sorts of rewards in choosing a low carb diet and lifestyle. People who embark on this journey frequently get more than what they expect!

Of course, no results are the same as we are all unique bodies and persons. HOWEVER, rest assured that you would definitely have a better well-being after adapting to a low carb diet. This is a guaranteed effect that *all* low carb dieters experience and have in common.

We are very glad that you have decided to make a lifestyle change with us. In this e-book, we will give you a perfect guide and ease your lifestyle and diet transition into a metamorphosis. In the next chapters, we will have a general discussion of the rules, strategies, and basic concepts related to a low carb diet. After that, we will give you *complete* recipes so you do not have to worry about what to do next in your lifestyle change.

These recipes are selectively handpicked and tweaked with your well-being and comfort in mind. These are very easy to prepare and contain ingredients that may be already available in your cupboard. Most of all, they are delicious and perfect for all seasons.

Let's get started!

CHAPTER 1: WHAT IS A LOW-CARB DIET?

The concept behind a low carb diet is simple: You have a "low" consumption of carbohydrates, or carbs for short. Any dieter understands that dieting is basically consuming less food and cutting portions. The low carb diet is similar to this traditional concept – eating less – but it has a little twist and varied results compared to other diets. Focusing on cutting carbohydrates provides a different dieting experience and results, something specific to low carb dieters.

Why do low-carb diets emphasize consuming low *carbs?* Why does it not focus on cutting calories or other food groups, instead?

To answer this question, first you need a basic understanding of the basic food groups and know where carbohydrates mostly fall in. The three elementary food groups are Go Foods, Grow Foods, and Glow Foods.

Carbohydrate-rich foods fall under the category of "Go" Foods because they give us energy to do daily tasks. Protein-rich foods are classified as "Grow" Foods because proteins contribute to muscle repair and growth. Lastly, fruits and vegetables are classified as "Glow" foods because of their high Vitamin C and mineral content that nourishes the skin and gives us a glowing, more beautiful, youthful appearance.

Take note that these categories are not *exclusive*. Anyone who reads food labels will understand that food consists of a combination of proteins, carbohydrates, and vitamins, among others. Some foods have the exception of being almost exclusive to one food group – corn starch, for example, is almost pure carbohydrate with a very few grams of protein – but nevertheless there is always a combination with a *dominant element* only.

This means that foods like meats, for example, are protein-rich, but not necessarily carbohydrate-free. The same is true with fruits. Some fruits have an incredibly high amount of carbohydrate, making your switch to fruit and vegetable snacks from bread and pastry snacks relatively pointless.

Once you start reading food labels, you will understand better what this food composition concept means. The important thing to learn here is not to generalize food items and categorize them into one of the three basic groups. Every food is unique; do not make stereotypes! We will illustrate this better in later chapters where *food you did not expect* from a low carb diet is absolutely recommended.

Right now it must be clear to you that what we are focusing on is *carbs*. Do not be allured by the fact that some foods are high-protein or fat-free. Always check if they are low in carbs. Even a high-protein food – like a triple-patty mega burger stuffed with cheese and high amounts of protein – does not guarantee that it is low in carbs. Food like this may actually contain a large amount of carbs compared to simple and obvious carb food, like rice.

Why choose a low carb diet?

Numerous diets and eating lifestyle are available at present that listing them down is a bit hard. There is a vegan diet, a low-calorie diet, a fat-free diet, intermittent fasting, a dairy-free diet, and so on. However, what makes the low carb diet different?

If you are planning to have diet and lifestyle changes, you must always know *why* you are choosing a particular pattern or regimen. Do not follow patterns "just because" nor choose arbitrarily. You must have a clear idea of the results that you are seeking to achieve and check if your goals fit what your potential dieting regimen has to offer. It is also very important to consult with your doctor first before making significant changes to your diet.

The main reason dieters choose a low carb diet is that it targets *fat loss*. If you want to grow muscle and achieve a "trim and cut" physique, this is a good option. Other diets such as low calorie and vegetarian will make it difficult to hit the gym and lift weights, for example, because this diet does not easily support such lifestyle (or bodily composition change).

Low carb diets will also not necessarily affect the amount of calories that you consume. If you love food and cannot bear to stand an empty tummy, then a low carb diet will suit you better.

How does a low carb diet work?

The science behind a low carb diet is easy to grasp. First, we need to understand what carbs are exactly and how do they work. What happens to our bodies when we decide to consume low amounts of carbs?

Carbohydrates provide energy. Of course, we do not always consume or burn the carbohydrates that we eat (thanks to the sedentary lifestyles promoted by advances in technology and civilization). More often than not, we have a *carbohydrate surplus* – the product of consuming more carbs than what our bodies actually need for energy synthesis – which our bodies will store eventually as *fat* for future use.

Icky, right?

What happens when we do the *opposite* – consuming less carbs to the point that our bodies do not get "enough" carbs?

We become *fat-adapted.* Our bodies will look for

something else to synthesize in order to make up for the carbohydrate deficit. In addition, you have guessed it right – our bodies will start to burn *fat* in order to maintain energy.

However, what about "decreased" energy levels? Isn't it true that carbs are responsible for providing energy to the body? Isn't it good for our health?

These are good questions to ask, and we have the answer. Your body will always adapt and change according to your lifestyle and environment. The transition to a low carb diet will undoubtedly be difficult at first, but eventually you will be fine and start feeling better.

In the next chapter, we will give you guides on surviving the toughest, first few weeks of the low carb diet. Lifestyle changes are all difficult at first, but if you get the proper guidance, the difficulty of making a positive change would not be so hard.

***

CHAPTER 2: - HOW TO LIVE A LOW-CARB DIET LIFESTYLE

Transitioning to a low carb diet from a relatively "high-carbohydrate" diet is not an easy thing; it is a challenge. It is a lifestyle change. It will almost drive you crazy.

All your life you have been eating starchy food and refined grains like rice, bread, pasta, potatoes, and cereal, then suddenly, you have decided to cut these food choices significantly. Wouldn't it drive you crazy if you cannot suddenly hang out in your favorite pizzeria? What do you say to your lover who regularly sends a box of cupcakes? Heck, what about the bag of potato chips that you always keep with you during movie weekends?

You may feel isolated and at many points in your life, you will be obliged to cook your own food or resist going out for dinner. Probably half of the groceries that you keep in your kitchen will disappear or you will need to replace them by something else. This is a daunting transition, but if you change your perspective, this can actually be a very good, refreshing thing.

Think of this as an opportunity to have a life-changing chapter in your life. A change in your diet is not just about what you put in your tummy. This will also likely affect the decisions you make, the thoughts in your head, and your daily activities.

It is crucial to get support from people around you. Are you switching to a low carb diet because you literally need to lose 100 pounds? Do not be ashamed to tell this to your friends and family; they will be happy for you and be glad to support you.

Low carb diet tips & suggestions

If you are fairly new to dieting, then take things slow. We suggest that you start dieting at a time when it is convenient because dieting causes a lot of stress, just like any lifestyle change.

Start your low carb diet during a vacation or during the time when your workload is not at its peak. If you have just retired from a job or finished school, you may just be at the perfect time to consider a low carb diet.

Avoid distractions. At many points in your dieting lifestyle, you may receive invitations to events, functions, and parties that will challenge your resolve when it comes to dieting. You can call these days "cheat" days, but do so only when you have no other option. Always say "no" whenever you can do so politely. Never let people control your own diet.

For best results, we also suggest that you couple your low carb diet with proper workout and exercise.

Consult a professional trainer and inform them about your chosen dieting regimen. Remember, diet and exercises are a couple that must always be compatible.

SUCCESSFUL STRATEGIES TO IMPLEMENT THE LOW CARB DIET

Everyone has his or her own coping strategies. Some methods work perfectly for others, while some do not give much result. However, it is important to get started with necessary advice.

These tips are basic strategies required to implement a low carb diet successfully.

1) Do not starve yourself. The low carb diet is not designed to slowly kill yourself. Never skip a meal when you are hungry, nor depend on sleeping pills to sustain an empty stomach to bed.

2) Take the low carb diet slow. Keep the transition gradual and do not surprise your body. Do not reduce more than half of your former carbohydrate consumption in the first week. Never attempt a next-to-nothing carbohydrate consumption. You will probably experience headaches, dizziness, light-headedness and lack of energy during the first few days, but this is normal. Get plenty of rest and do not attempt vigorous activities.

3) Read food labels. Take time to read nutritional facts and do the math. A low carb diet **contains 50-150 grams** of carbohydrates. As a starter, you may target 150 first. Be careful not to go way below 50 grams (remember dieting flu). Also, although the low carb diet is not restrictive on calories, make sure that you do not go beyond 2000 calories (for adult women) or 2500 calories (for adult men) every day.

4) Keep yourself inspired. Never, ever, give up on dieting and exercising just because you are losing motivation and inspiration. Visible results take months to achieve for some people. However, one thing is definite: any effort reaps results, no matter how small. Therefore, be patient and be consistent. In time, you will achieve your goals and get what you want out of the low carb dieting lifestyle.

5) Cook for yourself. Avoid eating out, unless you are visiting a restaurant that offers Paleo cuisine or a detox menu. These are rare to find, as menus like these are not a popular choice. The best place to find healthy food is in your kitchen, at your own hands. In the next chapter, we will give you delicious and exciting menus to try out!

CHAPTER 3:
LOW-CARB SNACK RECIPES

Snacking is an important part of any dieting regimen, contrary to the negative connotations attached to it. Eating snacks between meals keeps you from being hungry enough to eat more than you should in the next meal. It also keeps you energetic so you can do tasks without constantly getting hungry before or after an activity.

In a low carb diet, it is necessary to keep your snacks healthy and to mind the right portions and serving sizes. Snacks are also fun to prepare and come in countless variety. It will take the boredom out of strict dieting! In this series of recipes, we will teach you how to eat wisely in Paleo diet-inspired and detox diet-inspired snacks.

HOMEMADE BAKED CINNAMON-FLAVOURED APPLE CHIPS

We all love sweet snacks, especially during the summers and spring. These are seasons when fruit is delivered fresh, or when we can go apple picking ourselves.

Sounds exciting? We recommend you this recipe of

homemade cinnamon apple chips. Easy to make and nutritious, you can get tropical tastes in your mouth minus the guilt. This is also a bonus for chip-loving people who look forward to replacing potatoes in their diet.

Ingredients

- 2 apples (we recommend Honey crisp apples)
- 2 tablespoons cinnamon

Cooking Instructions:-

1. Pre-heat oven to 200 degrees and prepare a baking sheet with parchment paper.
2. Slice apples thinly to make crisp chips. Use a sharp knife to do this and be careful.
3. Remove the apple seeds.
4. Arrange the apple slices on the baking paper. Make sure that they are not overlapping in order to cook evenly with perfect crisp.
5. Gradually sprinkle cinnamon powder over the apple slices.
6. Bake the apple chips for approximately 1 hour. When brown, flip and bake for another hour.
7. Occasionally flip the apple slices until they are finally brown, dry, and crisp.
8. Enjoy this lovely snack! A serving of 30 grams has less than **25 grams** of carbohydrates. Tasty and guilt-free!

....

EGGPLANT JERKY SNACK

This second recipe is a delightful treat for people who love meaty, savory tastes. If you cannot wait until the next meal, satiate your taste buds with this healthy, low carb snack that will only give you **4 grams** of carbs.

We've used eggplants for this recipe. Like many other vegetables, eggplant carries next-to-nothing amounts of carbohydrates. You can eat almost as much as you want, just mind the sodium content and the calorie content of this snack, as they are not as low as the carbs in it. This recipe also requires marinating, so prepare this snack ahead of time.

Ingredients

- 1 ripe eggplant (about a pound)
- 3/4 cup olive oil
- 3 tablespoons balsamic vinegar
- 2 tablespoons maple syrup
- 1 teaspoon paprika
- Salt

Cooking Instructions:-

1. Slice a washed eggplant into thin strips. The thinner it gets, the crunchier and more satisfying

this snack would be. You can also cut long eggplants crosswise before making the strips.

2. Whisk together oil, vinegar, maple syrup, and paprika in a large bowl. Coat your eggplant strips using this mixture by placing and turning them with the ingredients.
3. Leave the strips soaked for 2 hours so that the eggplant strips absorb flavor.
4. Next, arrange the strips on baking sheets with parchment paper. Make sure that they do not overlap. Sprinkle with a pinch of salt.
5. Bake the strips on the oven's lowest heat setting for 10 to 12 hours. Turn strips occasionally to avoid burning or overcooking. They must be brown and crisp.
6. When done, place strips in an airtight container or zip lock bag. To absorb excess oil, place a paper towel around the strips.
7. Serve and enjoy this savory low carb treat!

ROASTED RED PEPPER POPPERS

This is another delightful snack for dieters who want to experience tangy flavors in their mouth without resorting to junk food or on-the-spot pizza delivery. If you love spicy food, definitely try this recipe.

Most spicy dishes sold outdoors tend to compromise the relatively carb-free ingredients (peppers) by mixing in "unhealthy" stuff like pita bread, cheeses, and god-knows-what sauces.

This recipe is safe from all of those unnecessary add-ons. Roasted, you can rest assured that this is also low fat and low-calorie. Did we mention that it only has **4 grams** of carbohydrate per serving?

This recipe is good for 12 people (perfect to make for a bunch of friends coming over) and takes only 30 minutes to cook and prepare.

Ingredients

- 2 red bell papers, large
- 6 bacon strips
- 1 piece small chicken breast, steamed
- red pepper flakes
- salt and pepper

Cooking Instructions:-

1. Pre-heat your oven to 375 degrees. For better taste, alight your grill prior to baking. This will add an elusive, smoky aroma to your papers after baking.
2. Chop your red bell pepper. Make large chunks of about 1 inch thick boats. Using two large bell peppers might produce fifteen pieces.
3. Drizzle the pepper chunks with olive oil. Season with salt and pepper.
4. Grill the peppers. After about 8 minutes, they will come out slightly charred. You may also skip this step and proceed to baking immediately.

5. Make strips out of your cooked chicken breast and produce about 12 small pieces. Do the same with the bacon strips and cut them lengthwise to produce a total of 12 pieces.
6. When done, let your peppers cool off. Prepare the snack by placing a strip of chicken meat in the pepper boats. Sprinkle with red pepper flakes.
7. Use the bacon to wrap the pepper boat nicely.
8. Bake your peppers for approximately 25 minutes, just enough time to cook the bacon. Grilled peppers will cook in less time.
9. Serve and have fun with the peppery taste!

CRISPY BAKED RADISH CHIPS

Ingredients

- 10 -15 large radishes
- nonstick cooking spray
- salt, to taste
- pepper, to taste

Cooking Instructions: - :-

1. Preheat an oven to 375 degrees.
2. Make very thin chips of the radishes by slicing them.
3. Place them of a cookie sheet, after sprinkling non-stick cooking spray on it.
4. Sprinkle salt and pepper on the radish slices.
5. Bake the radish chips for 10 minutes.
6. Turn them to bake for another 5-10 minutes.

7. *Take out when crisp.*
8. *Time may vary depending on oven and flipping time.*

....

EASY LOW FAT PARMESAN

Ingredients

- 1 cup zucchini, sliced
- 1 tablespoon parmesan cheese, grated
- becel topping and cooking spray (10 sprays or other light spray margarine)

Cooking Instructions:-

1. *Sprinkle non-stick cooking spray on a cookie sheet with aluminum foil.*
2. In a bag shake the zucchini, Becel and the parmesan cheese to coat it well.
3. Until the cheese starts to melt and brown, broil the cheese coated zucchini.
4. Serve warm.

....

UNFIRED CRISPY BAKED BEET CHIPS

Ingredients

- 4 beets, large, scrubbed clean
- nonstick cooking spray

- salt, to taste
-

Cooking Instructions:-

1. Preheat an oven to 375 degrees F.
2. In a food processor or with a slicing blade or a sharp knife or even a mandolin, slice the beet into as thin slices as possible, so that they become like potato chip.
3. Sprinkle nonstick cooking spray on a cookie sheet.
4. On the cookie sheet spread the sliced beets evenly and season with salt.
5. Roast the beet slices for 45 minutes to an hour.
6. Keep an eye on them to determine how crisp you want them.
7. Serve with sour cream or your favorite dip.

■■

BISQUICK CRUST BACON AND CHEESE QUICHE

Ingredients

- 8 slices bacon, cooked & chopped
- 1 small onion, chopped & sauteed
- 1 teaspoon garlic, chopped & sauteed
- 1/2 cup Bisquick (Heart Smart)
- 4 eggs
- 2 cups nonfat milk
- 1/8 teaspoon pepper

- 1/4 teaspoon salt (or Lawry's Seasoned Salt if you have it!)
- 1 1/2 cups low-fat cheddar cheese, grated

Cooking Instructions:-

1. Preheat an oven to 350.
2. Grease a pie plate or muffin tins with non-stick cooking spray.
3. In a medium frying pan, cook the bacon.
4. Depending on the type of pan and the type of bacon, if you are using turkey bacon, spray the pan with needed non-stick cooking spray.
5. Remove the bacon and add onion and garlic to the same pan.
6. Sauté them until they turn pink and translucent.
7. While this cooks, beat eggs and milk and whisk them together in a large bowl.
8. Chop the cooked bacons separately.
9. Add cooked onion, garlic, salt and pepper and the Bisquick.
10. Whisk it for 1 minute to make sure that there are no lumps.
11. Pour this Bisquick mixture to the greased muffin tin or pie plate.
12. Sprinkle cheese and bacon on top of it.
13. Bake until the top turns golden-brown.
14. As you insert a knife in the middle, it should come out clean.
15. If the internal temperature is measured to be 165 – 185 degrees Fahrenheit by a thermometer, the quiche should be ready.

16. Give it at least 10 minutes standing time, before cutting.

17. For Pie plate, it would take 40-50 minutes, for Muffin tin it would take 20-25 minutes.

18. It will make 2.5 muffin size quiches.

****

CHAPTER 4 : -
LOW CARB BREAKFAST RECIPES

The debate on the relevance of breakfast as a meal seems to go on forever. Some fitness guru advocate intermittent fasting, even one-meal-a-day eating, that requires a person to cut breakfast completely in order to achieve a limited "feeding window". Busy people, like students and employees, are always on the go and sometimes hardly find time to eat properly before starting the day.

Brunch lovers reason that three-meal-a-day eating is a matter of social convention. Let us not leave out grandparents, mothers, and schoolteachers who teach us that breakfast is the most important meal of the day.

So, how important is it to eat breakfast, really?

Each reason not to eat (or to eat) breakfast poses a specific argument that may be scientific, logical, or fallacious. Let's face it: each have acceptable points. In this e-book, we are not going to dig deeper into the issue of breakfast as a necessary meal nor provide an end to the debate. However, to implement a low carb diet successfully, we insist that you avoid experiencing hunger to better control your appetite and eating patterns. For this reason, we strongly recommend for you to have breakfast whenever you can and need to have it.

Besides, aren't breakfast recipes delicious and perfect to start the day? In this chapter, we will give you delectable dishes that are bound to make your day instantly.

APPLE BUCKWHEAT MUFFINS

Pastry for breakfast is common in many cultures and societies. The most popular pastry is probably bread, in all sizes, shapes, colors, and flavor. Pastries get high carbohydrate content from the amount of flour or grain used in it. It does not belong to a Paleo diet (Paleo is grain-free), but some pastry recipes can be part of a detox diet, which is still good for your health.

If you simply cannot let go of bread, or are trying to cut down on bread significantly, then this recipe is for you. We have prepared a low carb recipe with the same taste and nutritional content of a regular muffin. Yes! This recipe uses buckwheat flour for added nutrition and less carb content. One piece or serving contains only **29 grams** of carbohydrate. In your breakfast, you can have this 195-calorie treat side by side with a serving of salad or eggs.

Ingredients

- 1/4 cup buckwheat flour

- 1 tablespoon baking powder
- 1/2 tablespoon cinnamon powder
- 1/8 tsp salt (course)
- 2 eggs (large and farm fresh)
- ½ piece banana, mashed
- 1/4 cup honey
- 1/2 finely diced sweet apple
- 1/4 cup walnuts, chopped

Cooking Instructions:-

1. Pre-heat oven to 350 degrees. In a muffin tin, prepare four baking cups.
2. Whisk together flour, baking powder, salt, and cinnamon in a large bowl until the mixture is even. In another container, mix the wet ingredients – egg, honey, and banana – until smooth.
3. Combine wet and dry ingredients before folding in walnuts and apples.
4. Fill the tops of the lined cups with batter. Fill the remaining cups halfway with water.
5. Bake your muffins for around 30 minutes. Keep baking until a poking toothpick comes out clean. When done, let the muffins cool. Serve and enjoy a hearty breakfast muffin!

LOW CARB PUMPKIN SPICE PANCAKES

Pancakes are the classic breakfast food. It has been marketed and romanticized in movies and television shows as the delectable, homey, sweet and creamy delight. Breakfast in bed always involves pancake. When a couple united from a sweet night decides to eat out for breakfast, they go to pancake stores in their PJ's. Sweet. That is just how popular and appealing this soft and fulfilling food is. It also tastes really well with any beverage – coffee, chocolate, or juice. Wishing it is breakfast already?

Pancakes may be served plain, or with butter and maple syrup. Some go even fancier and add yogurt and fruit to the toppings. However, beware – pancakes can pack high amounts of calories and carbs if you're not careful with what you eat.

Regular pancakes sold in stores and cafes may not be friendly to a low carb diet, but your homemade, modified pancake can surely fit into your low carb commitment.

Tweaking some ingredients can significantly reduce calories and carb content. This recipe that we're about to share contains only **20 grams** of carbohydrate. Enjoy pancakes minus the guilt!

Ingredients:-

- 1 scoop protein powder (for reduced carb content)
- ½ cup shredded pumpkin (cooked)
- 1 tablespoon cinnamon powder
- ½ tablespoon baking powder
- 2 egg whites
- ½ cup uncooked oatmeal

- ½ cup + 3 tablespoons water
- Honey

Cooking Instructions:-

1. Mix dry ingredients in a bowl and sift.
2. When done, prepare a large blender. Mix the wet and dry ingredients. In a low setting, turn on the blender to mix the ingredients smoothly. Do not mix the ingredients for an extended period of time.
3. You may manually mix the ingredients, but using a blender will be handy if your shredded pumpkin is not so soft in texture.
4. Set the batter aside.
5. Spray a heated pan with cooking oil. Over medium heat, pour about a quarter cup of batter onto the pan.
6. Cook until bubbles emerge to the top and the edges look solid. Flip the pancake. You should have a golden brown color, but with a more golden accent.
7. When done, serve with a teaspoon of honey. This recipe makes three servings for you and your family to enjoy.

CHEESE AND HAM SCRAMBLED EGGS

If you love salty, rich food for breakfast, here is a delicious alternative to darling pancakes and muffins: cheese and ham with scrambled eggs. This a classic, once again, which has varieties that may not be good for your health, especially for old people. However, if you pick the right ingredients and tweak the recipe a bit, like the previous traditionally "non-diet" recipes, we can make this recommendable and enjoyable for low carb dieters.

This recipe is for a high-calorie breakfast excellent for those who need to be on the go. If you have a heavy job and won't have time to snack, choose foods that are high in calories, proteins, and fat, but not in carbs. This dish contains very little carbohydrates: **3 grams**. It has high protein content, good for those who want to build muscle.

With this breakfast, you will not easily feel hungry and keep your appetite satiated for hours. It is also easy to prepare!

Ingredients:-

- Butter
- 8 ounces of smoked ham, diced
- 6 fresh eggs
- 2 tablespoons of heavy cream
- Salt and pepper
- 1 tablespoon minced chives
- 2 ounces shredded cheese

Cooking Instructions:-

1. In a large bowl, whisk the eggs with heavy cream until frothy. Season with salt and pepper to your liking.
2. In a large, non-stick skillet, heat a tablespoon of butter. Be careful not to burn the butter and keep your flames low.
3. Sauté the ham in melted butter until it starts to brown.
4. Pour in the egg and cream mixture. Whisk with the ham and scramble over medium-low heat. Avoid overcooking to preserve soft texture.
5. Lastly, toss in the chives and cheese. Keep scrambling until the cheese starts to melt.
6. Transfer to a plate and serve hot! This delightful breakfast makes 4 servings.

MICROWAVE POACHED EGGS

Ingredients

- 1 large egg
- 1/8 teaspoon white vinegar
- 1/3 cup water
- salt and pepper

Cooking Instructions:-

1. In a 6-ounce custard cup mix white vinegar and water together.

2. In the same cup, break an egg and its yolk by pricking with a toothpick.
3. Cover it with a plastic wrap.
4. Cook for 1 minute in microwave or until it is done.
5. Experiment with the cooking time, depending on taste preference and microwave wattage system.
6. Remove egg from hot water immediately to stop cooking process.
7. Serve with salt and pepper.

BAKED HAM AND CHEESE OMELETTE ROLL

Ingredients

- 6 eggs
- 1 cup milk
- 1/2 cup all-purpose flour
- 1/2 teaspoon salt
- 1/4 teaspoon black pepper
- 1 cup cooked ham, chopped or 9 slices of any deli ham
- 1 cup shredded sharp cheddar cheese

Cooking Instructions:-

1. Preheat an oven to 450 degrees.
2. Grease a 9 x 13 baking dish or pan or lay butter paper on the dish.
3. Make a fluffy mixture of milk and eggs by beating them together.

4. Into this mix, add salt, pepper and flour.
5. Make a smooth batter by whisking properly.
6. Pour batter on the greased dish and bake for 10 - 15 minutes.
7. After 6 minutes interval, sprinkle cheese on top.
8. Bake for about 5 minutes, until cheese melts.
9. Roll the omelet and slice it to serve hot.

SAUSAGE GRAVY

Ingredients

- 1 lb pork sausage
- 1/3 cup flour
- 1 quart milk
- 1 dash pepper
- Pillsbury Grands refrigerated buttermilk biscuits

Cooking Instructions:-

1. After cooking the sausages in a skillet, drain all the remaining fat.
2. On the cooked sausages, sprinkle some flour to coat them well.
3. Cook these flour coated sausages for about 5 - 7 minutes.
4. Add the milk to it and cook it further to make it thick.
5. Sprinkle pepper and serve hot spreading over biscuits.

....

SCRAMBLED EGGS

Ingredients

- 8 eggs
- 2 tablespoons sour cream
- 1 tablespoon water
- salt & freshly ground black pepper
- 2 tablespoons butter
- 1/2-3/4 cup grated cheddar cheese (I use sharp)

Cooking Instructions:-

1. Beat sour cream, eggs and water in a medium size bowl.
2. Add salt and pepper to it to.
3. Whisk properly to make it fluffy.
4. Melt butter in a nonstick frying pan.
5. Add the egg mix to it and stir occasionally.
6. As egg cooks, add cheese.
7. When it reaches the desired consistency, serve with biscuits.

....

BREAKFAST BURRITOS

Ingredients:-

- 12 eggs, beaten
- 1 lb bulk sausage, cooked (or crumbled links)
- 1/2 cup chunky salsa (your choice of heat)
- 2 cups cheddar cheese, shredded
- 24 flour tortillas (you can also use whole wheat)
- Optional Ingredients
- 1 green pepper, finely diced (optional)
- 6 potatoes, shredded and fried until cooked through (optional) or 6 hash browns (optional)
- jalapeno, slices (optional)
- 1 (4 ounce) cans chopped green chilies (optional)
- 1 -2 garlic clove, finely minced (optional)
- 1 onion, finely diced (optional)
- 1 tomatoes, peeled and chopped (optional)
- 2 green onions, sliced with tops (optional)

Cooking Instructions: - :-

1. In a large skillet, scramble eggs, sausages and salsa.
2. Warm the tortillas for 20-30 seconds in the microwave.
3. Put 1/2 cup of the scrambled eggs and roll them burrito-style.
4. On a lightly greased cookie sheet, wrap the burrito and freeze it.
5. Freeze them even for a month.
6. When serving, unwrap them and microwave for 2 minutes until heated through.
7. Or you can also thaw burritos and wrap in a foil to bake for ten minutes at 350 degrees in the oven.

****

CHAPTER 5:-
LOW CARB LUNCH RECIPES

We can all agree on this: nobody skips lunch. It is one of the most important meals, allowing us to continue working hard for the rest of the day and make up for whatever we have missed during breakfast. Our bodies get the most fuel during lunchtime, mostly because we dedicate time and effort to make this meal happen. Depending on your schedule, lunch may be eaten a little earlier than noon, or mid in the afternoon. Nevertheless, one does not simply forsake getting a satisfying, tummy-filling lunch.

If you are on a low carb diet, getting diet-suitable lunch may be tricky. If you are working, one convenient option is to order a takeout at a fast food chain or have whatever your officemates are eating – pasta, rice, potatoes – foods that you are trying to avoid as much as possible.

Yes, it is going to be hard, but if you do not want to ruin your diet, make an extra effort and find a way to hunt a source for low carb lunch options. Do not even think about skipping lunch to attain a low carb diet! You just have to be creative. Once again, the easiest place to look for it is in your kitchen, and we're here to recommend recipes that will make your lunchtime enviable to non-dieters.

VEGGIE EGG SALAD

Salads for lunch are perfect. It has "class", good nutrition, and offers an explosion of fresh flavors in your mouth. If you are packing this low carb lunch with you to office or school, your friends will be impressed and see you as a health-conscious person, not a poor fellow who cannot afford to get "fuller" lunch.

This recipe contains vegetables and eggs, a perfect combo. Veggies are very low in calories and carbohydrates, giving you freedom to eat as much until you are full. Eggs, on the other hand, are protein rich and can keep you from feeling hungry for many hours.

This recipe is also simple and easy to prepare; time constraints are not a problem. You may also eat a double serving because this delectable delight only has **7 grams** carbohydrates. It is also low on calories: less than 150.

Ingredients:

- 3 tablespoons greek yogurt
- 3 tablespoons low-fat real mayonnaise
- ½ teaspoon ground pepper
- A pinch of salt
- 8 hard-boiled eggs, peeled
- ½ cup finely chopped (cubes or strips) carrot
- ½ cup diced cucumber (peeled and seeded)
- 1/4 cup sliced scallions

Cooking Instructions:-

1. In a medium-sized bowl, combine yogurt, mayonnaise, and salt. This will be your salad dressing.
2. Halve the eggs and discard four egg yolks (which you might save for future use).
3. Mash the eggs in the salad dressing until smooth.
4. Stir in carrot, cucumber, and scallions.
5. Let it cool. You may serve this salad with lettuce in order to add crisp. If you intend to pack this meal, do not mix right away the dressing and the vegetables for a fresher aroma.
6. Enjoy this low-carb, healthy and delicious treat!

CURRIED TOFU SALAD

The next gem on our list is a satisfying vegan recipe. Do not fret about it! If you love meats and savory food, we promise you this one does not have a bland taste like most vegan recipes. As a matter of fact, it is a vegan twist of a *chicken* recipe. Different ingredients, less carbs and calories, but with the same delectable delight! This curried tofu salad contains only **13 grams** of carbohydrates. If you had a muffin or pancake for breakfast (with significantly higher carb content), then you can make it up with this low carb diet-friendly recipe.

Ingredients:

- 3 tablespoons Greek yogurt
- 2 tablespoons low-fat mayonnaise
- 2 tablespoons mango chutney (prepared)
- 2 teaspoons hot curry powder
- 1/4 teaspoon salt
- Freshly ground pepper
- 14 ounces steamed tofu (drained, rinsed, and manually crumbled)
- 2 stalks diced celery
- 1 cup red grapes, sliced lengthwise
- 1/2 cup scallions, sliced
- 1/4 cup walnuts, chopped

Cooking Instructions:-

1. In a bowl, whisk together yogurt, mayonnaise, curry powder, and chutney. Add salt and pepper to taste.
2. When mixture is even, stir in tofu, celery, scallions, grapes, and walnuts.
3. You may serve this meal with accompanying lettuce and a slice of orange fruit. Have a great lunch!

··

CREAMY CHICKEN SALAD

Chicken recipes tend to overwhelm to the taste. Most dishes make you use tons of sauces and ready-made ingredients with additional carb content. It would be better to avoid recipes like this.

If you are sensitive to sodium content, non-salty popular chicken recipes cooked in broilers and steamers can get you easily bored.

This last lunch recipe, however, is a low carb treat that will bring out the sumptuous flavors from your chicken. You will not need sauces from the grocery store. We will teach you how to make them.

This chicken salad recipe releases the intense flavor of the meat without the use of so many additives. Only having **10 grams** of carbohydrates, this dish will keep you full, happy, and healthy.

Ingredients

- 2 pounds chicken breast meat, trimmed, and skinned
- 1 cup chicken broth (you can take used water from steaming chicken in other recipes)
- 1/3 cup chopped walnuts
- 2/3 cup low-fat sour cream
- 1/2 cup low-fat mayo
- 1 tablespoon dried tarragon
- Salt and pepper
- 1 1/2 cups celery, diced
- 1 1/2 cups red seedless grapes, halved lengthwise

Cooking Instructions:-

1. Pre-heat oven to 450 degrees.
2. In a large glass-baking dish, arrange chicken and pour in broth.
3. Bake chicken until cooked and no longer pink in the center.
4. When done, let the chicken meat cool and cut it into cubes. Set aside.
5. On a baking sheet, spread walnuts and toast them in the oven until lightly golden. This may take about 6 minutes. Let it cool.
6. In a large bowl, whisk sour cream, mayonnaise, salt and pepper, and tarragon. Toss in celery, grapes, the baked chicken and walnuts. Stir.
7. When done, chill in the refrigerator for at least one hour. Enjoy the blissful delight!

....

ROASTED CAULIFLOWER

Ingredients

- 1 head cauliflower or 1 head equal amount of pre-cut commercially prepped cauliflower
- 4 tablespoons olive oil
- 1 teaspoon salt, to taste

Cooking Instructions: -

1. Preheat oven to 425 degrees.
2. Cut florets (of the size of ping-pong balls) of the cauliflower discarding its core and thick stems and trimming its head.

3. Mix salt and olive oil in a large bowl and coat the cauliflower florets in it.
4. Spread them in an easy clean parchment baking sheet and roast for an hour or until golden brown.
5. Keep turning those 3 or 4 times.
6. Serve hot!

JALAPENO POPPERS

Ingredients

- 25 fresh jalapeno peppers
- 14 -16 ounces cream cheese
- 2 cups shredded cheddar cheese
- 2 (16 ounce) packages bacon

Cooking Instructions: - :-

1. Cut the peppers in half long-ways and remove its stems and seeds.
2. Fill the peppers with cream cheese.
3. Sprinkle cheddar cheese on top of the stuffed peppers.
4. Around each pepper half, place 1/2 slices of the bacon.
5. Bake for 10 to 15 minutes in a 450 degree pre-heated oven.
6. Take them out and let it reduce some heat.
7. Serve with cucumber salad.

....

CUCUMBER SALAD

Ingredients

- 2 cucumbers, very thinly sliced
- 1 red onion, very thinly sliced
- 2 tablespoons vinegar or 2 tablespoons lemon juice
- 2 tablespoons low-fat sour cream or 2 tablespoons yogurt
- salt and pepper, to taste (I like a lot of pepper)
- 1/2 teaspoon sugar
- 1 teaspoon chopped fresh dill

Cooking Instructions: -

1. In a large covered bowl, mix all the ingredients together.
2. Give it a good shake.
3. Cover it with lid and chill.
4. Serve cold.

....

HEALTHY BEAN SOUP

Ingredients

- 1 tablespoon olive oil
- 8 garlic cloves, minced
- 1 medium yellow onion, chopped
- 4 cups raw kale, chopped (be sure to remove the spiny sections, there won't be many, but those that remain will be tough)
- 4 cups chicken broth or 4 cups vegetable broth, divided
- 2 (15 ounce) cans cannellini beans or 2 (15 ounce) cans navy beans, undrained, split
- 2 (15 ounce) cans sliced carrots, undrained
- 1 (28 ounce) cans diced tomatoes
- 2 teaspoons Italian herb seasoning
- salt and pepper
- 1 cup chopped parsley
- shredded parmesan cheese

Cooking Instructions: - :-

1. Heat olive oil in a large pot.
2. Sauté garlic and onion in it until they turn pink and translucent.
3. Add in the washed and cleaned kale (with little droplets of water).
4. Cook them for 15 minutes by stirring until they turn into a lovely emerald green and wilted.
5. Add tomatoes, carrots, salt and pepper, herbs, 2 cups beans, reserving 1 cup and 3 cups broth (use vegetable broth if you are a vegetarian), reserving 1 cup.
6. Let it simmer for 5 minutes.
7. When the veggies are cooked, blend it in a food processor.

8. When it turns smooth, thicken it a little by simmering for 15 more minutes.
9. Ladle into bowls.
10. Sprinkle shredded parmesan and chopped parsley on top.
11. Serve with crusty bread.

■■■

FUSION AVOCADO!

Ingredients

- 1 avocado, pitted and halved
- 1 teaspoon soy sauce
- Garnish
- wasabi (optional)
- pickled ginger (optional)
- cilantro (optional)

Cooking Instructions: - :-

1. Using a spoon, loosen the skin of the meat.
2. Pour soy sauce over the avocado and scoop it out.
3. Using wasabi or ginger if you love the taste!

****

Chapter 6: -
Low-carb Dinner Recipes

Of all meals, dinner is considered the most socially relevant. Many people meet and greet during dinners – remember reunions, prom nights, anniversaries and celebrations? They usually happen over dinner.

There is just something elegant and whimsical about eating at night, in a place with fantastic ambiance and abound with elegance. Of course, the food has to match the festivity. If you are on a low carb diet, we guarantee that you can still enjoy a great dinner, especially if you are having it at home.

Our dinner recipes will make your evenings special and conducive to your commitment to low-carb diet. These recipes are guaranteed low carb and presentable for great dinners, for yourself or for other people.

Chicken Breasts with Green Chile

This delectable delight will bring joy to chicken lovers. This dish has a creamy taste paired with the juicy, sumptuous flavor of the chicken. An addition of green chili-almond spices it up and makes it exotic. Containing only **4 grams** of carbs, this meal will definitely be one of your low carb favorites.

Ingredients:

- 2 cups almond milk (unsweetened)
- 1/2 cup chicken broth (you may use leftover water from steaming chicken)
- 3/4 cup New Mexican green chilis; chopped
- 3 scallions, sliced
- 3 tablespoons toasted slivered almonds
- 1 clove garlic, minced
- Salt
- 6 chicken breast fillets (about 24 ounces)
- 1 tablespoon vegetable oil
- 1 tablespoon toasted sesame seeds

Cooking Instructions:-

1. In a saucepan, boil together almond milk, green chilis, chicken broth, almonds, scallions, two pinches of salt, and garlic. Reduce heat and simmer.
2. After 20 minutes, use an immersion blender to make a puree out of the boiled ingredients. You may want to let the mixture cool a bit before making a puree. Blend until smooth and set aside.
3. Prepare chicken by sprinkling it with salt. Heat oil in a large non-stick pan and cook chicken over medium-high heat. Cook one side until beautifully brown. This may take 1 – 2 minutes. Transfer to a plate and set aside.

4. In the same pan, bring back the first batch of cooked chicken and pour in your puree-sauce. Simmer in low heat and turn occasionally. Cook chicken until tender for about 4 to 7 minutes.
5. When done with the rest, remove from heat and present in a serving platter.
6. Pour remaining sauce over the chicken. Decorate with sesame seeds.
7. Serve this dinner with a smile. You can make this dish for six people. Perfect for evenings with guests!

Butternut Squash Soup

Rainy days and cold nights make us crave for warm soups that will soothe our noses and make us feel "snuggled" by the food. In times when you are having cough and colds, soups are a favorite remedy restoring health and feeling more comfortable.

If you love soups and find yourself craving one for dinner, out of the blue, then try this low carb recipe for butternut squash soup. It has a homey aroma and taste that will make dinners humbly intimate. Only giving you **10 grams** of carbohydrates, you can enjoy your soup to the last drop.

Ingredients:-

- 1 small to medium butternut squash (weighing approximately 1.5 pounds)
- 1 teaspoon canola oil
- 2 stalks chopped celery
- 1 diced onion
- 1 medium-sized carrot, chopped
- 1 teaspoon ground cumin
- 1/4 tablespoon ground chipotle chile
- A pinch of ground cloves
- 6 cups vegetable broth
- 1 teaspoon sea salt
- 1/4 teaspoon ground pepper
- 1/2 cup greek yogurt
- 2 tablespoons parsely, chopped

Cooking Instructions :-

1. Pre-heat oven to 350 degrees.
2. Prepare squash by cutting in half and removing the seeds. Place them on a baking sheet with the cut-side down.
3. Bake squash until tender when pierced with a fork. This may take about 45 minutes to 1 hour. When done, let it cool and scoop out the flesh.
4. In a large saucepan, stir in celery, carrots, and onion over medium heat. Lower heat and constantly stir until ingredients are soft.
5. Toss in the squash flesh, chipotle, and cumin to taste. Add cloves. Simmer ingredients with vegetable broth and keep the saucepan covered.
6. After 20 to 25 minutes, your vegetables will be cooked and tender. Let it cool a bit before proceeding to the next step.

7. Using an immersion blender, blend the soup and make a soft puree.
8. Season with salt and pepper. When done, transfer soup to a presentable dish and garnish with yogurt and a sprinkle of parsley.
9. This delicious recipe makes 10 servings and lasts up to 3 days in your refrigerator. Enjoy this delightful recipe!

....

PORK CHOPS WITH CREAMY MARSALA SAUCE

After an abundance of chicken recipes, we now present you a delightful pork recipe for our last dinner recipe. This has a sweet and salty appeal to the taste buds and has only **17 grams** of carbohydrates.

Ingredients:-

- 1/2 cup Marsala wine
- 2 teaspoons pure cornstarch
- 1/4 cup flour
- 4 boneless pork loin chops (about 1 pound), trimmed and thinned
- 1/4 teaspoon kosher salt
- 1/4 teaspoon pepper
- 2 teaspoons virgin olive oil
- 4 thin slices prosciutto (about 2 ounces), chopped
- 1 small onion, thinly sliced

- 3 teaspoons chopped oregano
- 3 teaspoons chives
- 1 cup non-fat milk

Cooking Instructions:-

1. In a small mixing bowl, bring together the Marsala wine and cornstarch. Set aside.
2. Sift flour in a shallow dish. Season pork chops using salt and pepper. Toss meat into the flour.
3. In a large non-stick skillet, heat oil over medium-high heat. Lower flames and toss in the pork chops. Cook until tender and browned on both sides. This might take about a couple of minutes per side. Transfer pork chops into a plate.
4. Add the prosciutto to the heated pan and cook. Stir constantly until brown.
5. Sauté with onion until softened and browned.
6. Add 6 tablespoons of the Marsala wine. Toss in the oregano together with the chives and bring to a boil.
7. Add a cup of milk and the previously reserved corn starch mixture.
8. Simmer and stir occasionally until sauce has thickened and reduced slightly.
9. Return pork chops to the pan and simmer.
10. Serve the pork lathered with sauce and garnish it with chives. Present your low carb dish with a smile!

BALSAMIC CHICKEN AND MUSHROOMS

Ingredients:-

- 2 teaspoons vegetable oil
- 3 tablespoons balsamic vinegar
- 2 teaspoons Dijon mustard
- 1 clove garlic, minced (or more!)
- 4 (4 ounce) boneless skinless chicken breasts, pounded to 1/4 inch thickness
- 2 cups small mushrooms, halved,or quartered if using larger mushrooms
- 1/3 cup chicken broth or 1/3 cup white wine
- 1/4 teaspoon dried thyme leaves, crumbled

Cooking Instructions: -

1. Heat 1 teaspoon oil in a nonstick skillet.
2. Separately mix the mustard, 2 tablespoons of the vinegar, and garlic in a bowl.
3. Coat the chicken both sides in this mix.
4. Transfer it to the skillet and cook for 3 minutes on each side.
5. Take it out and keep aside in a plate.
6. In the same skillet, add the rest of the oil and sauté the mushrooms in it for a minute.
7. Add the wine, vinegar and thyme to it.
8. As the mushrooms become deep brown, serve it with the chicken.

ZUCCHINI LASAGNA

Ingredients

- 2 1/2 cups zucchini, sliced lengthwise 1/4 inch thick (about 2 medium)
- 1/2 lb lean ground beef (I use 1 lb.)
- 1/4 cup onion, chopped
- 2 small tomatoes, cut up
- 1 (6 ounce) cans tomato paste
- 1 garlic clove, minced
- 1/2 teaspoon dried oregano
- 1/2 teaspoon dried basil
- 1/4 teaspoon dried thyme
- 1/4 cup water
- 1/8 teaspoon pepper
- 1 egg
- 3/4 cup low fat cottage cheese (or low fat or fat free ricotta)
- 1/2 cup mozzarella cheese, shredded (I use 8 oz. divided)
- 1 teaspoon flour

Cooking Instructions: -

1. Pre heat the oven to 375 degrees F
2. Separately cook the zucchini to make it tender and soft. Drain the fat and set aside.
3. Separately cook or fry the meat and onions similarly, to lightly brown the meat and make the onions soft and tender. Again drain the fat and set aside.

4. Then add the other 8 ingredients that come in the list next and bring them to a boil.
5. Reduce the flame or heat and without cover, let it simmer for 10 minutes, so that it is reduced to 2 cups.
6. Beat an egg separately in a bowl.
7. Add half of the shredded cheese cottage cheese, and flour.
8. Take a 1 1/2-qt. baking-roasting pan. Place half of the zucchini and half of the meat mixture at the bottom, then the cheese mix and the rest of the meat and zucchini on top of it.
9. Bake it for 30 minutes at 375 degrees F, without cover.
10. Bake for 10 minutes more with the remaining cheese sprinkled on top.
11. Give it a little standing time and serve hot.

SPINACH QUICHE

Ingredients

- 1 tablespoon vegetable oil
- 1 onion, chopped
- 1 (10 ounce) packages frozen spinach, thawed
- 5 eggs
- 3/4 lb muenster cheese, grated
- salt and pepper

Cooking Instructions: -

1. Preheat the oven to 350-degrees F.
2. Spray a corning ware quiche dish or a 9-inch pie plate with cooking spray or Pam.
3. Put a skillet on medium heat and sauté onion for 5 min or until browned.
4. Add the spinach to it.
5. Until the moisture is evaporated, keep cooking it.
6. Remove it from heat and let it cool.
7. In a bowl, beat an egg and mix the cheese to it.
8. Add salt and pepper to taste.
9. Mix the spinach and cheese mix together well.
10. Evenly spread the mix at the bottom and make sure that the top is even.
11. Bake it for 40-45 minutes or till the top becomes browned.
12. If a toothpick comes out clean after pricking in the centre, it is done.

GRILLED STEAK

Ingredients

- 2 teaspoons brown sugar
- 2 teaspoons garlic powder
- 2 teaspoons onion powder
- 1 teaspoon fresh coarse ground black pepper
- 4 (6 ounce) beef tenderloin steaks
- 1 tablespoon vegetable oil

Cooking Instructions:-

1. Preheat the oven grill to medium-high heat option.
2. Brush the stakes with oil.
3. Separately mix seasonings and brown sugar and sprinkle them on the steaks on both of its sides.
4. Press the seasonings to the steak.
5. Grill it on each side for 6 to 8 minutes.
6. When cooked through, serve with grilled and assorted vegetables.
7. To add crunch and to balance the meal, add a crisp mixed green salad.
8. Try the new Cracked Pepper A.1. sauce as it goes well with this steak.

MEATLOAF - LOW CARB

Ingredients

- Tomato Sauce Topping
- 1 (8 ounce) cans tomato sauce
- 1 (6 ounce) cans tomato paste
- 1/4 cup sugar substitute (such as Splenda)
- 2 teaspoons white vinegar or 2 teaspoons water
- Meatloaf
- 2 lbs ground beef
- 2 eggs
- 1/2 cup grated parmesan cheese
- 1/4 cup diced onion
- 1/4 cup red bell pepper, diced (roasted or fresh)
- 2 tablespoons chopped fresh parsley leaves
- 2 garlic cloves, minced

- 1/2 teaspoon dried oregano
- 1/2 teaspoon dried basil
- 1 teaspoon kosher salt
- 1/2 teaspoon ground black pepper
- 1/4 lb prosciutto, thinly sliced (optional)
- 1/2 lb provolone cheese, sliced

Cooking Instructions: -

1. Preheat an oven to 350°F.
2. Mix all the topping ingredients together, desired water to make it thin and set aside.
3. Mix eggs, herbs & seasonings, cheese, vegetables and the beef in a large bowl.
4. In a wax paper-lined jellyroll pan, place the meat mixture.
5. Form a 10x8-inch flat rectangle shape with the meat mix.
6. Place prosciutto slices and provolone slices on top of it.
7. Roll the meatloaf and seal its ends.
8. Into a loaf pan, place the seamed side down.
9. Spread the topping on top of the meatloaf.
10. Bake for1 hour 15 minutes in the oven.
11. Drain all the excess fat and let it rest for 10 minutes.
12. Serve fresh.

GREEN & YELLOW SQUASH 'LINGUINI'

Ingredients:-

- 4 green zucchini
- 3 -4 yellow squash
- 1 lb large shrimp, peeled & deveined
- 2 tablespoons olive oil, divided
- 4 garlic cloves, divided
- 2 tablespoons white wine
- 1/2 a lemon, juiced
- 2 tablespoons romano cheese, grated
- red pepper flakes, to taste
- 2 tablespoons parsley
- 1 tablespoon basil
- salt & pepper, to taste

Cooking Instructions:-

1. Cut off the ends of the rinsed and dried zucchini and squash.
2. Peel them lengthwise to make thin linguini/pappardelle-like strips of the zucchini and squash.
3. Continue only to take the crunchy part and as the seeds are seen, discard them.
4. Over medium-high heat, put a large skillet.
5. Add 1 tablespoon of olive oil.
6. Add the "linguini" zucchini and squash strips.
7. Sauté for about 1 minute.
8. Mince the garlic cloves and add half of the minced garlic cloves to the "linguini".

9. Add salt and pepper and remove them from heat.
10. Add remaining olive oil, remaining garlic, shrimp and stir for 1 to 2 minutes.
11. Add the red pepper flakes, basil, parsley, and lemon juice before the shrimps completely turn pink.
12. Add the "linguini", grated cheese and some salt and pepper to taste. Toss together for 1 to 2 minutes.
13. Serve hot with grated cheese and lemon wedges.

WARM STEAK-AND-MUSHROOM SALAD

Ingredients

- 1 1/4 teaspoons kosher salt, divided
- 3/4 teaspoon fresh ground black pepper, divided
- 1 lb sirloin steak (1 1/4-inch thick)
- 2 teaspoons olive oil
- 8 ounces mushrooms, sliced (any variety)
- 1 cup beef broth
- 1 cup dry red wine
- 2 garlic cloves, minced
- 12 ounces baby spinach leaves (12 cups)

Cooking Instructions:-

1. In a large heavy-bottomed skillet, heat oil over medium-high heat.

2. Season the steak with 1 teaspoon salt and 1/2 teaspoon pepper.
3. Cook it in the skillet for 8 minutes.
4. Turn when it is halfway done.
5. Remove from skillet, place it in a plate and keep warm.
6. Add more oil to the same skillet and cook mushrooms for 3 minutes.
7. Add the garlic, wine and the broth and cook it further for 10 minutes.
8. Reduce the broth to 1/2 cup.
9. Add remaining salt and pepper.
10. Remove a little broth mix for serving.
11. Divide the spinach among four plates.
12. Put mushrooms and sliced steak on top.
13. Drizzle the broth mixture on top and serve hot.

CHAPTER 7:
LOW CARB SIDE DISH RECIPES

Side dishes complement any meal, from breakfast to dinner. They are the add-ons that you purchase at a restaurant to add spice and additional flavor to your meal.

Don't worry – extra delight doesn't always mean excess calories and carbs. In this chapter, we have low carb recipes for side dish that you can always prepare when in the mood for a "bigger", varied feast.

SPECIAL CAULIFLOWER SIDE DISH

If you love vegetables and want to incorporate them to your meals, you will love this cauliflower dish. The flavors and the crunch of the vegetable will pop in your mouth and release delectable flavors. In addition, it only has **4 grams** of carbohydrates per serving!

Ingredients:

- 2 cups cauliflowerets, steamed until tender
- 1 tablespoon Greek yogurt

- 1 tablespoon real mayonnaise
- 1/2 teaspoon mustard
- A pinch of dill weed
- Salt
- Garlic powder
- 1/4 cup cheese, shredded

Cooking Instructions:-:

1. *Pre-heat oven to 350 degrees.*
2. In a small bowl, whisk together the yogurt, mustard, and mayonnaise. When even and smooth, add a pinch of dill, salt, and garlic powder according to taste.
3. On an ungreased 3-cup baking dish, transfer the cauliflowerets. Top this with the mixture in the bowl. Spread the shredded cheese.
4. Bake, the cauliflowerets, uncovered, for 5 minutes. The cheese will melt when the dish is done.
5. Transfer to serving plates and serve together with your entrée. This makes 3 servings.

TARRAGON-ALMOND GREEN BEANS

Green beans are popular ingredients for side dishes because they are crunchy, colorful, and mild in flavor. They are also diet-friendly – low in carbohydrates but generous in fiber. In this recipe, we'll share to you a side dish recipe consisting mainly of beans, with only **13 grams** of carbohydrates per serving.

Ingredients:

- One and a half pounds green beans; fresh and trimmed
- 1/3 cup green onions, sliced
- 1 garlic clove, minced
- 2 teaspoons virgin olive oil
- 1/4 cup balsamic vinegar
- Sugar
- 1 tablespoon minced fresh tarragon
- Salt
- 1/4 cup toasted almonds

Cooking Instructions:-:

1. In a large, water-filled saucepan, boil and cook green beans for 8-10 minutes. They must be tender after cooking. Drain and set aside.
2. Heat the saucepan and spray with olive oil. Sauté onions and garlic until tender.
3. In another saucepan, mix in salt and sugar, vinegar, and tarragon. Boil ingredients together with the cooked beans. When liquid is reduced by half, drain the beans and toss them to the onion mixture.
4. Cook and stir until heated through.
5. Transfer to a presentable, individual dishes and sprinkle with almonds. This recipe makes six servings.

Low Carb Italian Mushrooms Recipe

Italian cuisine offers high-carb delights. Pasta, pizza, sauces – certainly not that good for your low carb diet. However, if you really love the tastes from this wonderful country, you can still enjoy them by tweaking recipes into low carb dishes.

This final side dish recipe will bring back the good experience of Italian food without making you worry about carb content. This Italian Mushroom dish only has **6 grams** of carbs. Enjoy it as you want!

Ingredients:

- 1 pound medium mushrooms (fresh o canned)
- 1 large onion, thinly sliced
- 1/2 cup butter, melted
- 1 tablespoon salt
- 1 teaspoon onion powder
- 1 teaspoon sugar
- 1 tablespoon dried oregano
- 1/2 teaspoon ground black pepper
- A pinch of dried thyme
- 1/2 teaspoon dried basil
- 1 teaspoon dried parsley
- A pinch of celery salt
- 1/8 cup vinegar
- 1/3 cup olive oil
- 1 tablespoon water

Cooking Instructions:-

1. *For the Italian salad dressing:* In a small bowl, mix the dry ingredients. When evenly mixed, store in a container.
2. In a serving dish, whisk together vinegar, canola oil, water, and one tablespoon of the salad dressing dry mix.
3. *For the vegetables:* Meanwhile, in a three-quart slow cooker, arrange mushrooms and onions in a layer.
4. Mix together butter and the Italian salad dressing mix. Pour over vegetables.
5. Cover and cook for 4-5 hours or until vegetables are tender.
6. Serve in individual dishes with a slotted spoon. This recipe is good for six servings. Enjoy!

∎∎

CAULIFLOWER RICE - LOW CARB

Ingredients

- 1/2 head cauliflower
- 1/2 teaspoon salt (optional)
- Cooking Cooking Instructions :- :-
- Chop by hand or blend in a food processor to make the cauliflower come to a semi fine consistency.
- Steam it or you can microwave it to cook.
- Or you can simply sauté it with a little bit of butter.

- Make sure that you do not overcook.
- Low Carb Baked Spaghetti Squash With Garlic Sage Cream
- Ingredients
- 2 1/2 lbs spaghetti squash
- 3/4 cup heavy cream
- 1 garlic clove, pushed through a press
- 3 teaspoons finely chopped fresh sage or 1/2 teaspoon dried sage
- 1/4 cup parmesan cheese
- salt and pepper

Cooking Instructions :-

1. Pre-heat an oven to 400 degree Fahrenheit.
2. Bake a squash for 45 min, after pricking it thoroughly throughout the skin.
3. When it is tender, take it out of the oven and cool it a little bit.
4. Cut it into halves and scoop out its seeds.
5. With the help of a fork, pull the squash strands out from each side and put it in a bowl.
6. In a pan, heat garlic, cream and sage together.
7. Shift this to the squash.
8. Toss them together to slightly coat the squash.
9. Sprinkle salt and pepper to taste with parmesan cheese on top.
10. Serve hot and immediately.

EASY MASHED CAULIFLOWER WITH NUTMEG

Ingredients

- 1/2 head cauliflower, cut into florets (about 1 1/2 pounds)
- 1/4 cup butter
- 1/4-1/2 cup parmesan cheese, grated
- 2 -4 tablespoons milk or 2 -4 tablespoons cream
- 1/4-1/2 teaspoon nutmeg, grated
- salt
- pepper

Cooking Instructions:-

1. Steam cauliflower florets to make it tender.
2. Add all other ingredients. You can change the measurements as per your liking.
3. Mash it to make a consistency that you like.

LOW-CARB MUENSTER SPINACH PIE

Ingredients :-

- 12 ounces muenster cheese, sliced

- 2 (10 ounce) packages frozen chopped spinach, thawed and drained.
- 2 eggs
- 1/3 cup parmesan cheese
- 1 (8 ounce) packages cream cheese, softened
- salt
- pepper
- garlic powder

Cooking Instructions:-

1. Preheat an oven to 350 degree Fahrenheit.
2. Place 8 ounces of muenster cheese at the bottom of a 9 inch pie pan or a quiche dish.
3. Mix parmesan cheese, garlic powder, cream cheese, eggs, salt and pepper to the spinach, in a large mixing bowl. The must be drained out of all the water, as much as possible.
4. After mixing it properly, place it on the cheese slices in the pie pan and then place the rest of the cheese slices on top.
5. Bake it for 35 minutes.
6. After 10 minutes of resting time, serve it.

DEVILED EGGS DELIGHT

Ingredients

- 4 eggs, hard boiled

- 3 pieces bacon, cooked & crumbled
- 2 ounces cheese, shredded
- 2 tablespoons mayonnaise
- paprika (to garnish)

Cooking Instructions:-

1. Separate the egg whites from the yolks by cutting the eggs lengthwise.
2. Add the yolks with the other ingredients except for the paprika.
3. Fill the egg whites with this ready mixture and sprinkle the paprika on top.

···

TOMATOES PROVENCIAL -- LOW CARB

Ingredients

- 2 tomatoes
- 1 dash garlic salt
- 3 teaspoons fresh oregano (or 1/2 teaspoon dried)
- 1/2 teaspoon basil, fresh if available
- 1 teaspoon sesame seeds
- 2 teaspoons olive oil
- 4 tablespoons grated parmesan cheese or 4 tablespoons romano cheese

Cooking Instructions :- :-

1. Pre-heat an oven to 400 degree Fahrenheit.
2. Slice tomatoes in halves.
3. Line them up in a shallow baking pan with the sliced side up.
4. As the ingredients are ordered in the list, drizzle them on the tomatoes.
5. Bake it for just a few minutes in the oven or in the broiler, until the cheese is golden.
6. Use it as a side dish, or even as an appetizer.

■■

CHAPTER 8: -
LOW CARB DESSERT RECIPES

To all food lovers, this is probably the most awaited and exciting part: the desserts. No three-course meal is ever complete without a serving of dessert that makes the taste buds applaud the overall richness and tastiness of the meal. Desserts complement the main course and leaves a goodbye kiss on the palate.

They may seem like a luxury that low carb dieters cannot afford, but such is only true with some desserts. Sure, ice cream, caramel crème, and heavy pastries are out of the question, but there are still delightful recipes that are diet-friendly and low carb without compromising the goodness of the sweet taste.

LIGHT AND LOW CARB LEMON SQUARES

Take a bite of this delightful lemon square treats with a creamy, sweet, citrus flavor in the mouth. This is best served after a savory meal and eaten with a group, friends and family. Each serving only has **2.4 grams** of carbs, perfect for keeping a strict diet but a delightful experience with food.

Ingredients:

(Crust)

- 1 cup almond flour (ground fine)
- A pinch of sea salt
- 2 tablespoons xylitol (powdered)
- 1 tablespoon coconut oil
- 2 tablespoons unsalted butter, melted
- 1 tablespoon vanilla extract

(Topping)

- ¼ cup almond flour, sifted
- 1/4 cup xylitol, powdered
- 2 teaspoons sweetener
- 4 large eggs
- ½ cup squeezed lemon juice

<u>Cooking Instructions:-</u>

1. Pre-heat oven to 350 degrees. Line an 8-inch square baking dish with parchment paper.
2. For the crust: Whisk the almond flour, sea salt, and powdered xylitol in a large bowl. In another bowl, bring together wet ingredients: coconut oil, vanilla extract, and butter.
3. Mix wet and dry ingredients together until evenly combined. Arrange and press the crust dough evenly onto the bottom of baking dish.
4. Bake the crust until lightly golden, for about 15 minutes.
5. For the lemon topping: Whisk together almond flour, sweetener, powdered xylitol, lemon juice,

and eggs. Blend until smooth. Pour the topping evenly onto the cooked crust.

6. Bring them back to the oven and bake for about 15 to 20 minutes, or until toppings are gold in color. Refrigerate until cool.
7. Cut into bars and serve. This recipe makes 18 servings!

■ ■

LOW CARB FRUITY MOUSSE

Mousses are simply satisfying because of the soft texture and creamy taste. Do not worry about serving a delightful mousse for dessert. At only **9 grams** of carbs per serving, this fruity mousse will sweeten up your taste buds.

Ingredients:

- 8 ounces non-fat cream cheese, softened
- 1 tub low-calorie fruity soft drink mix, divided
- 1 cup skimmed milk
- 8 ounces whipped topping, thawed

Cooking Instructions:-

1. In a large bowl, whisk cream cheese and 2 teaspoons of the drink mix. Gradually add milk for an even and smooth texture.

2. Next, blend in the whipped topping. Keep whisking until frothy and smooth.
3. Refrigerate the mixture for 3 hours. You may also serve this mousse with a serving of fruit.
4. Serve in a cup. This recipe is a single serving for private enjoyment!

FLOURLESS BROWNIES

Most pastries are avoided in a low carb diet, but some make an exception.

This recipe for flourless brownies is a good addition to your diet, and has the same sweetness and chocolate goodness of a regular bakeshop-sold brownie. With only **3 grams** of carbs, you would not think twice about tasting this dessert.

Ingredients:

- 2 ounces of dark chocolate squares (unsweetened)
- 1 cup butter, unsalted and melted
- 1.5 cup sweetener
- 4 large fresh eggs
- 4 large egg yolks
- 1 tablespoon vanilla extract
- 6 tablespoons cocoa powder

Cooking Instructions:-

1. Preheat oven to 350 degrees.
2. In a saucepan, over very low heat, melt together chocolate and butter. Set aside for 10 minutes.
3. In a large bowl, beat eggs until frothy. Gradually add in the sweeter until mixture is fluffy.
4. Slowly and carefully, drizzle the butter and chocolate onto the bowl with eggs.
5. Mixture will become very thick. Gradually add in the cocoa.
6. On a greased 12x16 baking pan, evenly spread the batter.
7. Bake brownies for about 15 minutes. They should be done when tester comes out clean with moist crumbs, and the top of the brownies is puffed and has cracks.
8. Cool for an hour before cutting into 2-inch squares. This recipe makes 48 servings. Enjoy one square for dessert!

LOW CARB LEMON DESSERT

Ingredients

- 2 cups heavy whipping cream
- 1 scoop Crystal Light sugar free low calorie lemonade mix
- 8 ounces softened cream cheese

Cooking Instructions :-

1. *Add the lemonade mix to the cream to sweeten it as per your taste.*
2. *Use only one little tub of lemonade mix from the container.*
3. *Beat it together with the softened cream cheese.*
4. *Let it chill for 30 minutes.*

Low Carb Cheesecake Dessert

Ingredients

- 8 ounces cream cheese
- 1 cup heavy cream
- 1 cup cold water
- 1 (1 ounce) package sugar-free instant pudding mix (any flavor, I like white chocolate and cheesecake the best)

Cooking Instructions:-

1. *Mix all ingredients together in a bowl.*
2. *You can add sugar free jelly or fruits of your choice on top of it.*

Low Carb Pumpkin Pie

Ingredients :-

- 1 1/2 cups fresh pumpkin or 1 (15 ounce) cans pumpkin puree
- 3 eggs
- 3/4 cup Splenda Sugar Blend for Baking (see NOTE)
- 1/2 teaspoon salt
- 1 teaspoon cinnamon
- 1/4 teaspoon cloves or 1 3/4 teaspoons pumpkin pie spice
- 3/4 cup heavy cream or 3/4 cup light cream

Cooking Instructions: -

1. Add all the ingredients together in a large bowl and mix well.
2. Spread it into a well greased pie pan.
3. Bake for 30 to 40 minutes at 350 degree Fahrenheit.

Note - It is better not to use Splenda packets.

LOW CARB ALMOND COOKIES

Ingredients

- 2 cups almond flour
- 1/2 cup Splenda Sugar Blend for Baking
- 1/2 cup softened butter, replace with what ingredient (if you want cookie that holds together a little more easily replace 2 tablespoons of butter with 1 l)
- 1/2 teaspoon salt (if using salted butter, omit salt here)
- 1 teaspoon vanilla extract
- 1 teaspoon almond extract
- 1 egg (optional)

Cooking Instructions: - :-

1. Preheat the oven to 300 degrees Fahrenheit.
2. Soften the butter in an electric mixer blend.
3. Add all other ingredients on by one to mix together.
4. Make walnut sized balls from the dough.
5. Place them on an ungreased cookie sheet. This is because the butter and the fat from the almond flour will grease the baking sheet as the baking process start.
6. Bake for 5 minutes.
7. With a fork press down the dough lightly.
8. Bake for another 18 minutes.
9. Make sure that the cookies do not get browned but thoroughly cooked.

10. Give it a 5 minute standing time and then remove from the sheet.
11. You can drizzle unsweetened chocolate for a more festive look.

■■■

LOW-CARB CHEESECAKE

Ingredients

- 3 (8 ounce) packages cream cheese
- 3 eggs
- 25 (1 g) packets Splenda sugar substitute
- 1 tablespoon vanilla extract
- 1 teaspoon almond extract

Cooking Instructions:-

1. Preheat an oven to 350°F.
2. Mix all the ingredients together in a bowl, except for the eggs.
3. When they are mixed uniformly, add the eggs and beat into a creamy mixture.
4. In a greased pie pan pour or spread this mix.
5. Bake it for 35 minutes until golden brown and cracked around the edges.

****

CONCLUSION:

After sharing you recipes, tips, strategies and guides on how to adapt a low carb lifestyle, we hope that you are able to enjoy the prospects of the journey and become inspired to make a lifestyle change. Once again, we are telling you that changing your diet is not just about food, it is about who you are as a person and a unique individual.

The recipes that we have shared in this book are just few of the countless low carb recipes that are accessible and easy to cook, especially for home cooks. We encourage you to find more of them, through our guidance or at your own perusal!

The success of your low carb diet is always in your hands. In the end, it is only *you* who will decide what goes into your plate and how much of it you would eat.

Losing weight and fat is a dream of many people, but sadly, not all could make a complete lifestyle change in order to make this happen. *You* have an advantage over these people – you have gotten the guidance from us and you definitely know what to do now at this point. All you have to do is to carry out these strategies yourself.

Your success will be our success. Good luck on your lifestyle change and may you have a better health!

DID YOU ENJOY THIS BOOK?

I want to thank you for purchasing and reading this book. I really hope you got a lot out of it.

Can I ask a quick favor though?

If you enjoyed this book I would really appreciate it if you could leave me a positive review.

I love getting feedback from my customers and reviews really do make a difference. I read all my reviews and would really appreciate your thoughts.

Thanks so much.

Jamie Watson

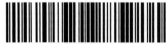
Printed in Great Britain
by Amazon